THOUGHT CATALOG BOOKS

How To Blow Like A Pro

How To Blow Like A Pro

And 25 Other Essays About Blowjobs

THOUGHT CATALOG

THOUGHT CATALOG BOOKS

Brooklyn, NY

THOUGHT CATALOG BOOKS

Copyright © 2016 by The Thought & Expression Co.

All rights reserved. Published by Thought Catalog Books, a division of The Thought & Expression Co., Williamsburg, Brooklyn. Founded in 2010, Thought Catalog is a website and imprint dedicated to your ideas and stories. We publish fiction and non-fiction from emerging and established writers across all genres. For general information and submissions: manuscripts@thoughtcatalog.com.

First edition, 2016

ISBN 978-1535049726

10 9 8 7 6 5 4 3 2 1

Cover photography by © www.gratisography.com

Contents

1

How To Blow Like A Pro: 10 Don'ts Of Giving Blowjobs

Phoenix Askani

After writing "Giving My First Blowjob", I realized how often fellatio is a topic of conversation in my life (SHOCKING considering the number of times I've done it on camera). So I'm back to talk more about BLOWEYS! I hate to toot my own horn here, but I've never had a complaint and I'm confident in my D S'N skills.

Recently I found myself wondering "How do you do this wrong? How do girls/guys give BAD HEAD? What are they doing, reading too many bad tips in *COSMO*!?" so I decided to ask several of my male friends (straight, bi, gay, and a couple porn performers) "What are a few of your least favorite things that girls/guys do when giving you a blow job? What are some moves you love?" My findings were interesting but not terribly shocking. I'm bearing in mind that not every girl is gonna have the same style and not every guy is gonna have the same preferences. Nothing wrong with that, to each their own! This list of the 10 worst things you can do during a blow job is based off of the most common responses from men, followed with my opinions, personal experience, and general advice on the subject. I also ran this by my friend Lexi Belle, winner of Best Oral Sex Scene at the 2013 AVN Awards for her scene in Massive Facials 4 (Elegant Angel Productions). This list has the stamp of approval from an award winning fellatio artist, so there's that.

Oh, and yes, I used caps lock as often as I felt like in this one, too.

1. Not Enough Spit

Hey, ladies? You know how friction can be uncomfortable when you're not wet enough? Yeah, well same goes for a penis. Not every guy likes a super sloppy blow job, but TOO DRY = NO GOOD. I'm huge into spit fetish, so spit strings, repetitive spitting, and drool basically dripping down from my mouth down my tits to my pussy are some things I'm into, but some people think that's excessive and gross, but oh well, it's what I like.

Do what you like, just make sure there's some oral lubrication going on. If you can and would like to deep throat, try inhaling through your nose and swallowing repetitively (like drinking a thick milkshake or whatever reminds you to swallow and open your throat – you're going for that GUH GUH GUH sound) and if you choke or gag on it a bit, you should be able to get a LOT of spit going. Obviously, keeping hydrated and having water at the bedside is also key, but that should go without saying.

Side note: If you know you can't deep throat without gagging uncontrollably and you've recently eaten or consumed alcohol or an energy drink, I would not advise trying to choke on that penis unless you both have a vomit fetish. I thought about making "DON'T VOMIT" it's own point, but I think that's sort of a given. If it does happen, not the end of the world, though probably a bit embarrassing. Any guy should be flattered you vomited from trying to get as much in as possible, though. That's some dedication. Yes, it has happened. Twice. It's not the coolest but you can totally recover from it.

Side note #2: Don't worry about the weird noises kissing, gagging, and sucking make. Those sounds just add stimulation to the male's mental state and boner. Slurp away.

2. No Eye Contact

Eyes are so, so, important during oral. Smile with them confidently. I'm not saying you have to stare deep into his soul the entire time, but if you don't look up at him once, he might think you're ashamed or not having a good time. Let the excitement of servicing his glorious tool show in your eyes! This segues into my next point…

3. No Sense of Enjoyment or Pride

I know some of you aren't huge fans of giving head (I can't understand your perspective but I can respect that everyone has different preferences) but at least try to look like you're having a good time and not doing it like it is out of obligation. I hope you ARE enjoying it, because I'd hate to hear anyone doing something they didn't want to do just to impress a guy. In fact, never feel pressured to give a blow job. If you don't want to and the guy whines about it, maybe you shouldn't be blowing that whiney child in the first place.

It's not exactly a huge turn on to suck a dick like it is the last thing you'd like to be doing at that moment. I'm heavily turned on by pleasing my partner, so GIVING is almost if not just as fun for me as receiving! I receive pleasure from doing everything in my power to see that he is having a great time while I'm on my knees. I think of it like I'm telling that penis a really fucking awesome secret. Try to only think about the cock in your mouth and how it makes you and your partner feel, what turns you on and enjoy being perverts together in that moment. Don't be afraid to express your enjoyment ver-bally, but your mouth should be busier sucking than speaking!

4. Too Much Teeth

I've met guys who didn't mind and are actually into a little bit of LIGHT teeth grazing on the shaft or even light nibbles on the balls... but again, NOT FOR EVERYONE. Most guys I've talked to about this subject have expressed a general fear and distaste for tooth to dick contact. Be careful, open up that jaw! I think this problem happens most often if the giver is in a rush or can't find a good rhythm. Take a short break, breather, or sip of water if you really have to, but try not to treat the dick like a toothbrush. You can and should treat it like lipstick though, sometimes it's fun to just smother it all over the outside of your mouth before you swallow it like a Creamsicle. I like to push it into the inside of my cheek (like you're putting your finger in your mouth sideways... not rocket science) and pushing it against the cheek wall (NOT BACK TEETH) and popping it out of my mouth before adding more spit, giving just enough time with my mouth off of the cock to add to the anticipation of it's return.

5. Not Enough Hands/Improper Hand Usage

Very rarely do I give a handy that doesn't turn into a blowie. I usually incorporate hand job moves and mouth moves together, using the hands as an extension to the mouth. Don't be afraid to grab firmly at the base and use some pressure. Don't forget the SPIT factor. Rotating the hand and changing pressure, speed, and length of stroke is always good too. Mix it up, and read the responses! If you can wrap two hands around the penis, stacked, and still get your mouth on the head — move up and down rhythmically while twisting the hands in opposite directions, clockwise and counter-clockwise. Don't hold it like you're afraid of touching it and don't suck it like your mouth is trying to run away. Make sure the grip is firm but don't rip it off, and keep the spit going whether or not your mouth is on the head! For a good pornoxample of hand usage and pretty much every point covered here, check out Bonnie Rotten's good ideas during her POV blow job in Facial Overload #3 (Evil Angel Productions). She nails the eye contact as well, for certain.

The hands rule doesn't just apply to the genital area, while licking the shaft or jerking the cock with one hand, you could be caressing their stomach, chest, hip area, and inner thighs as well, increasing the overall area of sensation. If the guy is standing while I'm kneeling, I like to grab their legs for a some face-fucking then gasp for air, slow it back down for a bit, bringing my hands back up to the base and stroking again. There's nothing wrong with touching yourself simeltaneously too, if you just cannot contain the enjoyment you're receiving from giving pleasure!

6. Don't Forget the Balls

Again, all back to personal preference, and in some cases, pubic hair shaving preferences. If there's a forest down there, I don't blame you if you're not in a rush to shove the sack in your mouth… a little bit of ball hair won't kill ya, though. If they're clean and the dude LIKES ball play and you don't mind going squirrel status on those nuts, you're both in for a good time. Maybe you'll even progress to the taint or anus with your tongue if that's something you're both comfortable with. At the very least, touch the balls with your hands! I just covered it but for emphasis INCORPORATE YOUR HANDS, whether it's a light tease or a firm grasp or tug, give them some attention! There are men who are very sensitive when it comes to their jizz holding manlyhood, so definitely communicate or pay attention to how they react. Proceed with caution. Don't hurt their balls… unless they ask you to. Those guys exist, too.

7. No Initiating

Do you make the move on your own? Did you tell him you want to blow him? Did you unbutton his pants and rub it outside the underwear in anticipation? Does every blow job you give begin with a request for one? If you're making out for like 45 minutes and he finally starts pushing your head down towards his crotch, you can probably reason he is passively asking for some licky-dicky. Don't be scared to initiate! I don't believe you should always have to, and I'm very appreciative of men who go down on me first, but it doesn't have to go the same way every time! Sometimes you're in the passenger seat on the way home from Vegas and you know you can help keep the driver alert and awake by offering a little lip service. Chances are, your good deeds will be rewarded. Initiating also shows confidence and lets the man know that you're willing and comfortable with him.

8. Don't Rush It

Don't rush like you can't wait for that to be "enough" for him. Don't look over at the clock. Don't think about the errands you have to run. Don't ask him "Is that enough?" or "Is this good?" Be cognizant and move forward accordingly. Go with that blow flow and be present. Remember, foreplay is important! It's like pre-heating an oven for a pizza. Everyone involved needs to get warmed up and the tease is hot! Unless it is a morning quickie beej before work, take your time and have fun with it before rushing into sex. Avoid deliberately sighing because you're just over it and want him to hurry up and cum. He'll sense your attitude and it definitely won't help him get off any faster. Short breaks are even cool for people into kinky play – take it out and slap it on your tongue, touch elsewhere, work the balls (back to 5&6), a little tease & denial or hair pulling… whatever floats your boats and keeps the penis erect.

9. Too Repetitive

If I come across a porn scene in which I see the girl bobbing up and down with a sad turtle mouth and no variation, I'm like, "NEXT!" Don't be fucking BORING, for crying out loud. Like I said in #5, change up the hand use, or even put them behind your back for a minute and pretend you're aggressively bobbing for apples. I like to challenge myself. How low can I get down on this thing? I don't mind gagging or running short of oxygen at points, it just makes me wanna go harder. Move your lips. Make out with it. Circle your tongue around the head. Lick from the base to the tip. Spit on it and grab it firmly and look him in the eye with dat hunger. Variation is good, but don't jump and skip around too quickly – use moderation. For emphasis, PAY ATTENTION TO REACTIONS AND/OR COMMUNICATE. I know I'm listing all these pointers, but the biggest pointer is to NOT THINK ABOUT IT LIKE A TECHNICAL/MECHANICAL PROCESS, but rather a sensual experience. Don't check off things in your head as you go, but if you know he has a favorite move, like the two hands or ball-sucking & licking, mix it in, go back to some strong sucking for a while, alternate again, move on. If you get bored in one position, change it. Ass up and on your knees if he's laying down, kneeling if he's standing, 69ing, laying down face-up when he's standing if you can take a lot in your throat… there are so many options!

10. Don't Run Away When He's Gonna Burst

This is a tricky one. If your partner/boyfriend/fuck buddy whatever is tested, and you want to swallow his juice, open that mouth up wide and look at him while he empties life source down your gullet. I KNOW NOT EVERYONE LIKES TO SWALLOW OR BE CAME ON. Cumed on. JIZZED UPON. Whatever. Not every guy can expect every girl to be down with that, either. Oh, and guys – informing us is nice. I like hearing when a guy is ready to cum, but sometimes I ask for it because I can tell he's getting close because I know that facial expression all too well. Not everyone turns into a perky baby bird when that time *cums*… too much? Okay. Maybe you're down for it to get on your face or tits but not in your mouth or not swallowed. That's all fine and good! If you are strongly opposed to something, communication in advance isn't the worst idea. If a dude is about to bust on your face and you suddenly do a tuck and roll, you're gonna fall off the bed, he's gonna cum all over the pillow… it may be easier to let it land and ask for a clean towel or some baby wipes after. I like to feel prepared, so obviously I keep some sort of wiping mate-rial on the nightstand next to my hydration station.

Bonus Tip

(for playing more than "just the tip"): If you've never tried coconut oil as a lubricant, you're in for a treat. Be warned though, coconut oil is known to break down latex, so if you're having safe sex during oral or after, be sure to use a latex free condom or rinse off the coconut oil so it doesn't break down the condom. I personally like to put some coconut oil in my mouth so it melts and drips down as I begin to suck and incorporate it into the blowjob. You can also warm it with your hands and do the double hand handjob method in #5 using spit and coconut oil to make it slippery and fun. This is a great time to try the stacked hands if you can, turning them in opposite directions or switching which hand is on top, while using your tongue on the head and frenulum.

HAPPY SUCKING!

2

How To Receive A BJ In 6 Simple Steps

Anonymous

Now I'm fairly certain that most of us have come across articles teaching us 'How To Give a Blow Job' and learning how much or how little to use your tongue, to keep your mouth wet (blah, blah, blah), even how to resist our natural gag reflex in order to successfully deep throat—oh joy! But what seems to be lacking from this topic, is one on how to actually receive a blow job...

If you're a boy who moans about women hating giving blow jobs then you can only blame yourself. I've varied from loving giving boyfriends blow jobs to point blank refusing based solely on their reactions.

1. First and most importantly, do not shove our heads into your groin. When asking friends what we most HATE about giving blow jobs, the most repeated response was the head shoving. Shoving our heads down to your crotch as sign language for 'Please can I have a blowjob?' or shoving our heads when we're already down there is really not enjoyable. Don't make me gag with your cock in my mouth—that's not sexy.

Let us take control. If you want us to take it deeper, faster, slower then TELL US, don't force us.

2. Don't just stand there with your hands on your hips like your some kind of sex Superman. Touch us! I personally quite enjoy a head massage whilst giving a blow job. If you have conveniently lanky arms then play with our tits during—for most girls nipples are a turn on spot! Sex in any form is an intimate experience and as it's difficult (but hot) to maintain eye contact whilst giving/receiving head using your hands is a good way to create intimacy.

3. Respond positively and vocally. Let us know we're doing a good job, gasp if we lick that oh-so-sensitive tip, and tell us how great that feels. We want to know exactly how amazing we are at blow jobs—it's good for the ego.

4. Hygiene. I know it's obvious but please, please, wash before we go down there. If it smells, it's gross, and we won't be going back there in a hurry. Obviously there are exceptions; if it all happens rather spontaneously or you're slumming it in a festival then it can't really be avoided.

5. Warn us before you cum. There is nothing more disgusting than choking on a load of cum you weren't aware was 'coming'. Also, ask us if we're ok with you coming in our mouths. Whilst many assume that there is the simple choice of spit or swallow you could actually just cum elsewhere—in a tissue, on our tits, anywhere but our mouths. An ex boyfriend once came on a load of revision notes and a library book next to his bed in a bit of a fluster. (Whilst this wasn't ideal it was funny in a oh-my-god-this-is-awkward-way and I actually appreciated him not making me swallow it.) No woman should ever feel pressured into swallowing cum.

6. Return the favor! Be chivalrous, if I go down on you I expect you to go down on me or use your hands. Heterosexual porn scenes usually involve the girl giving the guy a blow job followed by intercourse. Rarely does the man return the favour. This is SO not okay. Good sex involves satisfaction for both.

Following these tips will not only make oral sex a more pleasurable experience for your partner but also a more regular one for you!

3

Ladies, Here's 5 Quick And Dirty Tips On Sucking D*ck

Sean Jameson

These 5 blow job tips will show you exactly what you need to do if you want to give your man incredible and memorable oral sex. In fact if you do it right, then you can sure that he will happily return the favor!

1. Build Up To The BJ—Oral Sex Foreplay

Often you may find yourself making your way straight to your man's crotch from simply kissing him. This is all fine and good. But men actually enjoy foreplay too! This is an blow job tip that many don't realise. While men love quickies, foreplay makes their orgasms feel a lot stronger and more enjoyable than just 30 seconds in your mouth.

So instead of just ripping his pants off and taking him straight into your mouth, start off slower. Try lowering your hand to his crotch, outside of his trousers and gently massage him through his trousers. When you get his trousers off, stimulate around his legs and groin area before you finally take him into your mouth. This BJ tip where you build up to oral sex will literally have him begging you to speed up…perfect for building anticipation!

2. Don't Forget About Your Hands

Just because you are using your mouth to give your man a BJ, it doesn't mean that you should leave your hands idle and doing nothing.

Instead you should be using them to massage, rub, stimulate and caress around his member. So do pay some attention to his testicles. When you are grabbing and rubbing them, just make sure to be very careful though. Many who first hear about this blow job tip get a little excited and accidentally squeeze too hard and just end up hurting their man.

So remember to be soft and gentle!

3. Make It Wet

Of all five blow job tips in this article, making your blowjob wet is the easiest but possibly the most important. Making it wet for him means that it's going to feel a lot more luscious and sensual which means that his orgasm will feel a lot stronger and more enjoyable when he does reach orgasm.

If you naturally produce a lot of saliva, then you are off to a great start at making your oral sex a wetter experience. But if you don't (or if you want to make it even wetter) then you should consider using flavored lube on him. Alternatively, if you want it to taste even better, then try whipped cream or even some syrup. I cover this in much more detail in the oral sex instructional video along with the most important blow job techniques that you should be using on your man.

4. No Teeth!

Many women want to learn oral sex tips on how to make their BJs better for their man. But very few look for the things they should *avoid* doing during it. This is critical if you want your man to have a good time.

The number one thing that you should avoid when giving your man head is…using your teeth.

His penis is obviously very sensitive, so even accidentally grazing it with your teeth can be incredibly painful for him. And for most men, pain is a turn off. If you find that it's difficult to avoid accidentally grazing his penis with your teeth, then a great technique is to wrap your lips back around your teeth so that they have no chance of coming into contact with his sensitive bits.

5. Variation

You can know all the techniques in the world, but if you don't vary them and actually try new blow job tips, then your man is going to get bored. And we all know that boredom is a massive relationship killer. You need to be constantly trying new things with your man in the bedroom if you want to keep him satisfied. Keep what works and forget about what doesn't.

4

Inner Monologue Of Someone Not Getting A Blowjob

Jimmy Chen

Really, these Emily Dickinson poems are quite touching. Been trying to "dive into" celibates this time in my life, the alliance of the unlaid I suppose. *A death blow is a life blow to some*—wait, what *is* she talking about? Also have that red snapper in the fridge which I should make with some potatoes and leek—cook that down with a nice Chardonnay, a flick of paprika, and try not to cry into my skillet.

Oh, and there's that Thelonius Monk rare session take I need to explore, could listen to that on repeat while I eat my sad snapper. I like how jazz is basically attention deficit disorder on Adderall, and how men who listen to it seem irrevocably indignant about their abstruse taste. Maybe if I name drop Thelonius Monk at a party I might get someone's number, some girl impressed by absurd classist things. This is how things seem to work.

It's Saturday night, the night of wet sloppy blowjobs all across this baby-making-but-not-tonight world. From bar bathroom stalls, to limousine rides, to college dorm rooms, to plush douchey condos, to that abandoned Pontiac on cinderblocks covered in leaves in someone's backyard. Seems like blowjobs are happening all over the place: spunk flying slo-mo in glorious arcs, wads hitting tonsils like boxing speedballs, the emphatic male redundancy of *oh, yeah baby*. Jesus, I just got really depressed.

If you think about it, a blowjob is kind of crazy—not in a psychiatric or morally qualitative sense—I mean like the ponderous somewhat overwhelming logistical measures it takes in getting a complete well-minded stranger to voluntarily put your potentially unwashed hence "dick cheesed" penis into their mouth and "bob" their head in unison with rugged manual jerks until, if they are considerate, you blow your baby glue. Seems insane.

I'm actually kind of glad I'm not getting a blowjob now, like I'm shortlisted for the Nobel Peace Prize for not subjecting well educated and politically empowered women to my dank splooge. Have some chicken salad or tofu; that's all the protein they need. I'm a good person who enjoys refining his sensibilities reading Emily Dickinson poems about death. I hear she was a lesbian. Good for her.

And the Nobel Prize goes to mister Chen, for making dinner alone—dropping in half a stick of butter since he's feeling masochistic and fat—and eating it to not Thelonius Monk but a crass late-'90s comedy with reoccurring titty shots only obliquely tied to the narrative. For wanking out his juvenile violence to an aptly paused frame, and leaving innocent women out of it. What a great guy.

5

On Blowing A Zucchini

Jimmy Chen

As a feminist, I'm one to try to understand the female condition, put myself in their shoes, or—since we're inserting things—put an anthropomorphized phallic vegetable in my mouth and perform fellatio. I was curious about how it felt on the "giving" end, the sensation distributed along my tongue, the swollen wordless joy against the insides of my cheeks, the minor strain of my jaw down my neck, the thoughtful rhythm I employed slowly disappearing downward along my spine, the odd yet intuitive impulse to close one's eyes. Oral sex's recipient is nothing but *ooh* and *aah*, swamped by the boringness of vowels, head cocked back squinting into the fireworks between synapses. To venture into the world, the mind, of the subordinate "giver" is more interesting, maybe.

The idea of sexual orientation is—for a rather conventional straight dude—imperative. I am straight, and highly skeptical of the notion that everyone is somewhat bisexual. Girls can "accidentally" make out at a party, and not only is the universe is still in tact, it is made a little more awesome. A dude's ding dong in my umber yahoo and the world as I know it, via my end, would end. I would never blow a dude, yet somehow to blow a zucchini seemed, and still seems, reasonable; like the latter doesn't make me gay, simply curious and rather comprehensive in my approach. Perhaps some codependent part of me wants to understand how these women feel. Despite the feminist ringtone "empowerment," the blowjob seems just a little humiliating, more so than cunnilingus, which is just earnestly trying to pick up a raw salmon filet without using your hands or teeth. Maybe I'm projecting. Maybe porn—the evil that men do, under the sheen of its aesthetic glory—has changed us.

Before you think me obsessed, I did not venture out and buy a zucchini for this. I was in my condo, in bed I believe, wishing someone would blow me. This train of thought eventually, somewhat inversely, led me to want to blow something myself. I mentally listed phallic objects in my condo whose girth and length seemed penis-like. A cucumber (semantically embedded with cum) seemed more fitting for a black dude, and due to our deeply institutionalized imperialism of the West, I imagined blowing a white male, still the leader of our world. "Holy crap, I think there's a zucchini in my fridge," I thought, half-way out the bed towards the kitchen. And there it was, lying there in the fridge's light bulb's cold glow, all nonchalant and studly. I picked it up, my heart racing a little bit.

Wash your vegetables, my mother always said, so I did, dutifully moving my hands over it like a handjob. "Slut," I thought to myself. I brought it back to bed, laid on my stomach, and blew it. Going through the charade and light narrative was important. I didn't just want to stand in the kitchen blowing the zucchini. Sex, like a painting or photograph, is never about the mere incident, but rather, the preceding and subsequent chronologies which host the emotional volition—however empty, grim, compulsive, or self-hating—of such an act. In bed, my big boy was sitting up, legs spread, as my head bobbed up and down coaxing our future children into my mouth. The zucchini was missing the mushroom-like head, and I wondered if I had any mushrooms in the fridge. This was getting complicated. I needed to go to Whole Foods.

It's harder than you think. (I'm speaking to straight dudes here, you ladies and gays are doing just fine.) You quickly notice your jaw, and the taut contraction of neck muscles required to retract your mouth open. Teeth is another thing. The entire psychological logic of the blowjob as "naughty" surrogate vagina à la unconditional acceptance crumbles at the sensation of teeth, unless you're a sick bro with some omnivore or cannibalism fetish. However "natural" the act supposedly is, you will come—*please*, that is far from a pun—to discover how absurd it is to place a relatively large object in one's mouth, and to move back and forth for an extended amount to time, either denying or succumbing to the gag reflex, until genetic matter is promoted to an appetizer or dessert. God gave us penis and vagina, a holy trinity without some third wheel, and we gotta come along and put dicks in butts and mouths. Perhaps with each transgression, we are complicit in our own existential defeat. No matter what hole is filled, its conscious host still perceives an emptiness grander than its body.

Did I end up eating the zucchini is a reasonable question. And if so, did I castrate it into little pieces for a quick stir fry. But if I didn't, out of some ambivalent emotional attachment, did I throw it away or compost it. Did I, had this little enterprise been real, spit or swallow. The answers are these: No, I did not eat it, as it was too "personal" by now; and no, I did not compost it, because a zucchini will have little trouble degrading in a landfill, despite what these eco-fascists think. And I would have swallowed, because my love, or rather my need to be loved, is bottomless, save the pit of my lonely hungry stomach.

6

A Gay Man's Guide To Giving The Best Blowjobs

Adrien Field

Straight girlfriends often ask me with the same wide-eyed mystification about tips for giving head. They figure, rightly so, that there's no better resource than a gay man to dispense advise on how to orally please another man. As both givers and receivers of head, we are intimately aware of the mechanics involved.

The first time a guy came in my mouth, I felt a surge of pride, as if I had just completed a marathon and that was the prize waiting for me at the finish line. In fact, that's precisely how you should think about giving a blowjob—it's not a sprint to the end, it's more of a slow, steady pace to climax.

The blowjob is a handy tool in any sexual enthusiast's arsenal. Sometimes you just don't want to get pounded but your man is next to you, and he's hard, so what are you going to do? You could give him a desultory handjob, but that's the sexual equivalent of going to In-N-Out and only getting a bag of fries: nice as a side, but hardly a full meal. In these instances, the blowjob can be a stand-in for full-on penetration. No man has ever complained about having someone go to work on him while he lies back floating in a cloud of warm pleasure.

Now it's cliché but true that they don't call it a job for nothing. For the receiver, it's like a paid vacation, but for the giver it's equivalent to working overtime. Your jaw can get tired, you might choke a few times, gasping for air, and frankly you can get bored if it's going on for a long time. The trick is to develop a good technique so that he comes before you get lockjaw. So while the dick has to be hard for a blowjob, a blowjob doesn't have to be hard. Here are some foolproof tips for getting him off.

Ideally he's already hard, as there's nothing sadder than a life-less dick in the mouth. Both the giver and receiver have to be in the mood, though frankly a man is never not in the mood for a blowjob.

Get it wet. Spit on it. Pour a bottle of champagne on it. Just make sure you've got ample lubrication happening and your work will be much easier.

Don't spend all your time and devotion on the head, make sure you're loving on the entire kielbasa. Place one hand on the base of his dick and the other on his balls. You can give them a gentle tug, and massage the perineum (please don't make me explain what this is).

Your lips should be covering your teeth and you can move your tongue to massage the shaft. He's not going to cum if you're just licking his dick daintily as if it were a candy cane on Christmas. You don't have to deep throat, but at least get your mouth to meet the hand you have on the base of his shaft. Use the patented pump and twist ™ technique with your hand as you bob up and down.

Blowjob is a bit of a misnomer. A more accurate description would be suck job—use your mouth like a Hoover to create a vacuum of pleasure. If you have to come up for air, make sure to continue stroking. Maybe do a sexy hair flick and let him see your tits.

All men want to thrust into your face—this hip motion can make him come faster as he controls the intensity. The key here is to open the mouth, relaxing the jaw and breathe through the nose. If you can master breathing without gagging while he does this, it's the quickest way to get him to come.

You'll be able to gauge the pleasure by his face. If his eyes roll back in his head and he emits animalistic groans of delight, then you're doing it right. If he's watching you intently as if you were trying to build a computer out of Legos on his lap, then your technique is off.

As for spitting or swallowing, it's all a matter of preference. It feels great to cum inside a mouth, but after the party's over do whatever you want with the confetti.

7

Blow Job Lessons From My Best Friend's Dad

Adrienne West

Of all the memories I have of being 19 and having an affair with my best friend's dad, the one that I think about most often is the first blow job lesson he gave me. He loved oral, both giving and receiving, and he wanted to make sure I knew how to enjoy both.

For most guys truly good head is a once in a lifetime thing. If you know how to do it right a guy will remember you for the rest of his life.

He said this to me before we really started anything serious, we were in his bed after sex just talking, and he was going on about the value of good oral.

The idea intrigued me greatly, most of my friends hated giving head—or at least hated doing it for more than a few minutes. I was interested in approaching the whole thing a bit differently. I didn't want to hate doing something the guy I was with loved. It seemed like a source of endless friction. I wanted a kind of explosive partnership that was much more intentional about mutually being the best for your partner than passively hoping for their infallibility.

I don't like the middle of the road, if I was going to do something at all, I wanted to do all of it—be the best at it, or at least take it to it's farthest end and experience it fully. Why be a bear at all if you're not going to be a grizzly? When I was younger I denied myself cream and sugar for a long time, until I learned to love the taste of coffee without it, and now I'll never need cream or sugar. When something is good for you, you just have to learn how to love it.

All this to say, he wanted to give me blow job lessons, and I was ready to be a very good student. I knew that not every man was going to like what Steve liked, but I figured it would be easiest to adjust from guy to guy when I at least knew one really well. Like how learning your second foreign language is a lot easier than learning your first.

One afternoon I was packing an overnight bag to meet Steve at his lake house when he texted me:

You'll learn about blow jobs tonight. Come very hydrated.

I grabbed a water bottle and sipped drank it on the short drive to the lake house. When I parked I saw he was waiting for me. Seated on the porch with his back against one of the cedar posts, reading something, or pretending to read at least while he waited for me. He looked so handsome like that.

"How's school?" he asked. I laughed, it was funny to him that I was a student, that I was so much younger than him. It turned me on as well—and I couldn't tell if it was his pleasure at the situation or my own curiosity about someone with a few decades of experience on me.

He poured us some wine inside the house and I drank nervously—he always made me nervous, it was part of his charm. Even when we just talked he stood closer to me than a person normally would. It intimidated and excited me. I took a step back and hopped up on the counter, he stood between my legs and kissed me, wrapping his arms around me and pulling me into him tightly, making the kiss more urgent than casual. I wanted to lay on the counter and feel his weight on top of me right then, but I knew that wasn't his plan for the night.

"Can we just have sex first?" I asked, a bit breathless from his advance and finding an irresistible urge inside me to get a quick fix in.

"No..." He moved from kissing my mouth to my neck. "It's good to delay gratification a bit. It makes it better, you'll see." It was impossible to see how he could be right, but all I could do was try to persuade him through *other* means. Maybe if I started to rub his cock he'd be overcome by the same lust that was making my brain fuzzy. I reached my hand down and felt him, he was definitely hard. But he merely grabbed my hand and deposited back on the counter.

He made us cook dinner then. I've never seen anyone look so sexy while dicing vegetables but I couldn't think about anything else. Everything was sex. Chopping vegetables was sex. Stirring a sauce was sex. Watching his mouth while he drank wine was sex.

I was quiet while we ate. I preferred to stare at his mouth and hands and fantasize about the place on my body I'd put them rather than make polite conversation. As if he could read my mind he was patient with my silence, the corners of his mouth turning up when he caught me lost in thought, my eyes focused on him.

I placed my dishes by the sink after dinner, expecting him to tell me we had to clean up first, too. But I felt his mouth on the back of my neck, his arm reaching around me stomach and pulling me backwards into his body. He reached one hand forward and cupped me between my legs and I felt myself coming undone with anticipation.

"Let's go upstairs."

He brought me to his bed where he sat, and I kneeled in front of him. He looked so loving when he looked at me.

"You should always start playfully. Don't be too quick at it. You should act like all you want in the world is the guy to cum, but you're not in a big hurry to get it over with. Run your tongue around the edge of the head, especially on the underside. And then when you start taking it in your mouth, hide your teeth behind your lips."

I did all these things for a moment, it felt a bit disjointed but I noticed his hips writhing a bit and it became more natural, more fun. It wasn't my first blow job, but it was my first time trying to do something specific, or even trying really hard at it.

I tried to remember what he said and smiled internally (something someone told me about coming off as having a good time once) before running my lips up and down his shaft, pausing at the tip to lick my way around it and then taking more of it in my mouth, swirling my tongue around it when I slowly pulled it out.

He stood up then, and steadied my head between his hands while he helped me get the rhythm down, pushing himself in and out of my mouth.

He stopped me while I was catching my breath and lifted my face with a few fingers under my chin. "Men want to admire your face while you're doing this. You look so good with my cock in your mouth," he pushed himself back in my mouth, watching me intently as he pushed himself in and out again. He must have been right, I'd never seen his face look like this before. He was so focused, even if just to memorize the moment.

"Curl your tongue, make a snug bed for my cock." "Cup the balls. Don't play with them separately, but as a unit." I followed his instructions.

All of this is, I guess, considered a warm-up. When he's really ready to start Steve told me coordination is important. I needed to move my mouth in sync with my hands so it felt like one thing was happening instead of two separate things.

"See if you can catch your breath while you still keep it in your mouth. Just relax your lips over just the head and pull on it, breathe through your nose."

I tried this and it was unexpectedly easy—but probably because I knew he was expecting me to stop and test this out.

"You can always ask a man what he likes you to do. I like to get deep inside. I want to feel your throat. It mimics sex, but it's more relaxing. And more exciting." I was nervous about this part, but the good kind of nervous, because I knew I'd be happy I did it. And he made me feel very safe. I took him back in my mouth and allowed him to move his hips forward while holding me in place. This is where I discovered my own trick, when I resisted my urge to back off, I found my mouth suddenly filled with my own saliva. My body produced more of what I needed when I pushed it to the edge, and I suddenly had lube for my hand to run up and down his shaft.

He wrapped his hand around mine and showed me the speed and firmness he liked, keeping his other hand on the back of my head to keep us in sync, every few moments removing our hands and hitting my throat with his cock.

"When I speed up, it means you're doing a good job. I'm getting closer." He told me, as he speed up our routine.

He told me that some guys like you to go until completion and others just want to warm up for sex, they want the act of finishing inside you, it's a primal instinct. He was of the latter persuasion.

"When a man says he's about to cum, keep doing what you are doing, and if he is guiding you, let him take over. He knows what he needs."

I removed my hand from his cock and ran them up and down his thighs to signal that I was willing to do this. I looked up at him as I suddenly felt salty pre-cum in my mouth. He was looking at me intently, pumping in and out of his mouth. I struggled not to move even though his groans were really turning me on. Finally I felt him break rhythm and push himself deep inside my mouth, depositing his semen down the back of it. It was always a bit difficult not to gag with the surprise of a guy cumming in your mouth, but since it was so far back, it was easier as it was already being swallowed by the time I realized what was happening.

He fell back onto the bed behind him. "Goddddd Adrienne, you're already very good at this."

This wasn't the last blow job lesson, we usually practiced before sex from then on, but they got quicker — which I took as a compliment.

8

What It Feels Like To Get Your D Sucked

Ryan O'Connell

Many of my girlfriends have asked me the question, "What does it feel like to receive a blowjob?" They tell me that they yearn for a penis just so they can experience it themselves. I, for one, understand this completely. I can't imagine clocking in countless blowjob hours without a guarantee that you're going to get yours. I like giving them mostly because I like penis. As a gay man, it's sort of in my job description. But I'm not sure how pumped I would be if a blowjob wasn't promised to me in return (unless of course, I loved the dude and we were in a relationship. Then you don't keep score.)

But even though you *should* return the favor, it doesn't mean you're going to *want* to, especially if you're with someone you don't care about. And that's okay! Because above all else, giving a blowjob is exhausting. I'm not just saying that to be cute because oh my god, they don't call it blowJOB for nothing, right?! No. I'm just saying that giving someone a blowjob is an amazing gift. It's better than paying for dinner at Buca di Beppo, it's better than filling someone's gas tank up, it's better than paying for the movie *and* popcorn. It's "Let me move my mouth up and down on something jarring while using both of my hands feverishly. Let me sweat in really unattractive ways and be in a really vulnerable position." Even though blowjobs are less intimate than something like anal sex, they're still a sexual act that requires trust and understanding. Like you could be really bad at giving head (it's really hard) and you want to make sure you're with someone who won't judge you. You want to be with someone who's willing to correct years of bad technique because they care! (Unless it's a one night stand type of situation. Then there's no need for the Sting and Trudie Styler kind of communication. Just do your thing, let him do your thing, and get out.)

You know what's the worst? When you're giving head and someone pushes your head down further so you choke on their dick. It's like, "Can you not? I know you want to feel like you have a huge penis right now but it really hurts and makes me feel degraded. So cut it out!" I always get uncomfortable when someone's going down on me and I look up and they're staring at me dead in the eye. I know it's supposed to be sexy or whatever, but it just kind of freaks me out.

Oh, right. I guess I should finally get to the whole "what it feels like to get your dick sucked" part of this article. I'm sorry, I didn't know I had so many feelings regarding this subject. OK, so getting your dick sucked can feel one of three ways: Amazing, painful or like nothing at all. Seriously. I once was with someone ages ago who would go down on me and it would feel like air. I would have to check to see what he was doing down there because it felt like nothing was happening. In a way, I guess this is a good thing. If someone's bad at giving head, it's best that it feels like nothing rather than painful hell. But it still weirded me out. How can you put a mouth on a penis and have nothing happen??!!

The best part of a blowjob for me is not when they're going down on me, but when they come up for air and start jacking you off. They've lubricated your dick so well with their mouth that it's created a pleasurable waterslide (BTW, too much saliva is a bad thing. I once was with someone who drowned my penis and it made my dick so sensitive that I would have spasms if he touched it. Quell embarrassing!) Anyway, the moment a guy comes up and starts jacking me off, it feels amazing. Kind of like I'm going to pop/explode/whatever. The actual sensation of a mouth on your penis feels exactly like how you would think. However, it's the mixture of saliva and what you do with your hands that makes it go off the charts.

One thing you should know about how it feels to get your D sucked? It's a fine line between pleasure and crippling anxiety. As you may know, all men aren't created equal. Some take 5 minutes to cum (bummer) and some take 30 (exhausting bummer). If a dude is taking too long, it's kind of crazy how mental he can become. He feels terrible that you're working so hard and there's still no orgasm at the end of the blowjob tunnel. Of course this anxiety makes it impossible for him to cum, and then it becomes a blowjob aborted. With most sex stuff, most of it is all mental.

Blowjobs are fun. Blowjobs are stressful. Blowjobs are major work. Blowjobs are the kindest gesture. But they're really not all that complicated. In fact, I would kill to know what it feels like to get eaten out. Or just what it feels like to have a vagina in general.

9

'S' Is For Swallow: A Blow Job Alphabet

Jillian Paulson

We've discussed the A to Z of sexting before, and you guys liked it so much I thought we should tackle another sexy topic- the blowjob. So many words have been spilled about this (sometimes) simple sexual practice, but as a certified blowjob pro I think my words carry just a liiiiittle more weight.

A is for Alcohol

Don't drink too much pre-blowjob because you might vomit on his dick. I'm just saying this might have happened to some- one I know...someone who may or may not be me. Booze- heavy nights out and BJs don't mix!

B is for Breath Control

There's a reason they call a blowjob a job. You have to figure out how to breathe, when to swallow and how not to gag when you deep throat. It's work!

C is for "Can I Have a Blowjob?"

Which is what he's going to ask you for the rest of your life if he's into your technique.

D is for Deep Throating

Practice makes perfect!

E is for Eye Contact

Make it. Porn basically primed men to require eye contact while you're doing the job.

F is for Fun

Sometimes, blowjobs are a chore. I totally get that. But they're also a fun opportunity to practice your skills and make your dude freak out. Act like you're having a great time (or actually enjoy it yourself!) and it'll enhance the experience for both of you.

G is for Grip

A tight-ish one is best. Make a fist around the base of the dick and move it up and down just a little in time with your sucking. Easy-peasy and works like a charm.

H is for Hands

Use them! Don't just suck and lick the dick; add a little grip with one of your hands and try different movements to mix things up.

I is for Ice Cream

It's a stupid women's magazine trick, but pretending that dude's cock is an ice cream cone you just can't get enough of works every time.

J is for Jerking Off

I once fooled around with a dude who could only cum if you blended a blowjob and a handjob—like, just good ole junior high jerking off. It was not my ideal situation, of course, but he was really into it and the contrast between a warm, wet blowjob and then a handjob really worked for him. Don't knock it 'til you try it!

K is for Know Your Zones

It's not all about the dick, you know. Pay attention to the balls, to that little spot where the head meets the shaft, to the "taint" area (ew, I hate that word) and please the whole crowd!

L is for Lubrication

Get the good spit way back in your throat because its thick consistency lubes everything up so much better.

?M is for Main Event

I usually prefer to keep the blowjob strictly in the foreplay section of sex, but sometimes it's fun to get down on my knees and surprise a dude with a middle-of-the-day, no strings attached blowjob.

N is for No Rushing

A slow, teasing blowjob just enhances the excitement and pleasure.

O is for Orgasm, duh

Some dudes can bust in a few minutes from a good beej and others take awhile. Some prefer it as foreplay and others just really want a BJ. Whatever floats your boat.

P is for Pre-Cum

Don't be surprised to see a pearly little bead of pre-cum when you're giving a great BJ! I think pre-cum is sexy, and when it happens during a BJ I just flick it with my tongue.

Q is for Quote

"If we perpetually gave men blowjobs, we could rule the world." –Samantha, Sex and the City

R is for Return the Favor

If you go down on him for an extended period of time and give him a deliciously good BJ, he needs to return the favor for you! If he doesn't, withhold the blow.

S is for Spit or Swallow?

I don't know anyone who spits out jizz post-blowjob orgasm. Do you? I've always swallowed.

T is for Teeth

Be careful you don't slice up the soft, sensitive skin of a dick with your molars! Usually, dudes can deal with a little scraping and if they whine about it, they're probably being a baby. Some guys even like a little tooth action. Just be careful.

U is for Unique

Do your thing! Don't just go through the same boring motions over and over, even if they are effective. Mix it up and try new things to put your own sexy little twist on a blowjob.

V is for Vibration

It's basically proven that guys like it when you hum a little bit while you're blowing them. You can even use your vibrator on a low setting on their balls.

W is for What Not to Do

Don't suck or lick on the head of his dick right after he cums. It's a little too sensitive immediately post-orgasm and it might hurt.

X is for X-plore

I'm just saying that dudes really like butt stuff. I'm JUST SAY-ING that sometimes a little rimjob enhances the blowjob!

Y is for You're Doing Just Fine

I'll never forget my first blowjob. I was 16 or so and though I'd read a ton of Cosmo articles about BJs, I didn't actually know how to give one. You just gotta go for it and listen to how the dude is reacting, then change things up based on that. You can do it! I have faith in you! Most dudes would say any blowjob is better than no blowjob.

Z is for Zzzzzz

Which is what men tend to do after they have a really good orgasm. Which you provided. If you're annoyed with your boyfriend and want him to shut up and take a nap one afternoon, give him a blowjob and then he'll pass out.

10

10 Crucial Things He Wants You To Know Before You Give Him Head

Anonymous

1. It's not a race

Some guys can come as soon as a mouth gets within like 1 second of their cock and, I mean, I guess that makes your task that much easier! No matter what, though, sucking him off is not a race. It should be something you enjoy doing and that he enjoys having you do. Don't do it if you don't enjoy it because, first of all, fuck that, and secondly it's going to be a terrible blowjob if neither of you wants to be there. A good blowjob is never quick. You have to savour the penis, like an excellent boy steak lol.

2. Using your hands is cheating

There are people out there who think that you can get away with giving head if you just put your mouth on the tip from time to time and jerk him off for the rest. But that's not a blowjob. A blowjob is mostly mouth work and you use your hands as an additional flourish to give that extra sensation when he's least expecting it. Rather than using your hands throughout, try bringing them in only occasionally as a grace note to your performance. Using your hands the whole time is cheating.

3. Teeth

NO.

4. Caress him

It's easy to think that head jobs are all about the penis, but actually there's other stuff around there, too! Feel up on his stomach, around his legs, thighs, feet, nipples. Put your hands up on his neck. This will certainly amplify all the work you're doing and it will make him feel good, and it will make you feel powerful knowing that you can make him feel this way.

5. Touch yourself

Don't forget to touch yourself, too. There are plenty of guys out there who want to feel worshipped, who want you to worship their fucking cocks to the exclusion of your own pleasure. Fuck that—but actually. Touch yourself! Plus, he will like knowing that you sucking him off makes you want to touch yourself. THAT is a turn on.

6. Be really, really fucking excited to get his D in your mouth

Sex is always about enthusiasm. Do you want to be in that bed/backseat/bathroom stall with him? If you don't, the sex WILL be bad because all you can think about is the end. A good blowjob is an enthusiastic blowjob. That doesn't mean you need to be moaning and ooh-ing and aaaaaaah-ing at every slurp, or slurping at all because this is real life not porn and humans do not come with sound effects. But being excited does show him that you really like sucking him off and doing so is just as good for you as it is for him.

7. Simply Bobbing up and down for 10 minutes is so boring

I mean he'll come, yeah, because physics, but it won't be an earth shattering load. Be inventive, ladies and gay dudes!

8. Do things with your tongue

Speaking of being inventive, try doing different things with your tongue! You don't have to be "sucking" the entire time. Even just licking like a lollipop can feel good and hands down for every second his dick is not in your mouth and you're doing other things, teasing him in other ways, I guarantee you he's dying for you to put that D back in your mouth and he doesn't know when you're going to and aaaaaaaaah the anticipation!

9. Not all guys like their balls played with

Just a gentle FYI before you go pulling and crunching.

10. See what he responds to, then keep doing exactly that

The best blowjob tip you can ever receive is to do some stuff, see what he responds the most to and keep doing that. Every guy likes something different, and if you can figure out what he likes without him saying anything, you'll have him, well, by the balls.

11

18 Dudes Describe What It's Like To Get A Bad Blowjob And What Makes It So Terrible

Lisa Woods

1. "Like getting socks on Christmas Day."

—Darrel, 24

2. "There's really nothing more tragic than a bad blowjob. There are a lot of reasons it could be bad but, in the moment, the realization that you'd rather be changing your oil than receiving the blow job that's being thrust upon you is enough to make you question your whole life, your sexual orientation, whether you left the stove on, everything really."

—Mark, 26

3. "Usually when it's bad, bad, bad it's related to teeth being used. I'm not sure how a girl can't tell when she's banging her teeth with some dick, I'm really not. I mean, you brush your teeth, right? You know when the brush is hitting your teeth, you can feel it. I don't understand this."

—*Scott, 22*

4. "I've only had one blowjob that I would say was terrible and it was because she had a tiny, elfin mouth. Like, I had soooo many fantasies about that cute mouth and when the moment came it was like sticking my dick in a pencil sharpener."

—*Isaiah, 27*

5. "It never fails, girls who say they love giving head the most are always the worst at it. In my experience, the ones that don't like it have learned how to get it over with quickly but girls who 'love it' just like lick on it and stare at you and shit. Please don't just stare at me and lick my dick. This isn't a staring contest."

—*Marvin, 21*

6. "Some blowjobs hurt but some have just been annoying. I hooked up with one girl who was obsessed with not getting hair in her mouth and would stop every few seconds to like make sure there wasn't any getting in there. I'm like, my genitals are mostly covered in hair, maybe it's the male body you actually don't like. Anyway, a blowjob has to have flow and stopping every few seconds to sort of complain about hair destroys the experience."

—*Josh, 25*

7. "A lot of girls do not understand how a penis works at all.

They don't know where it's sensitive or where it isn't sensitive. I've had a few girls just lick my shaft over and over and then look at me and ask 'do you like that?' I mean, no, you aren't doing anything that feels particularly good. This woman was literally 30 years old. There's no hope for her ever being good at it."

—Bret, 28

8. "A little enthusiasm is pretty necessary. The worst ones I've had were given by girls who seemed to be trying to seem bored so that I'd ask them to stop. Wish granted!"

—Howard, 24

9. "Okay, I'm going to give your readers the real deal. Ladies, if you don't swallow or do something dirty with the cum then we're going to be disappointed. Jacking us off in your hand or on our own stomachs after a joyous blowjob is just about the most high school thing ever."

—David, 27

10. "I don't mean to be mean because I will always appreciate a girl being willing to blow me but there have been a few that were really ruined by the girl absolutely not listening to what I said I liked and I don't even mean anything weird. I just mean basic stuff like 'use your hands.'"

—Nathan, 22

11. "I dated one girl for a few months and the first time she gave me head I literally wondered if she'd ever done it before. I understand first times are always nervous so I thought things would get better. They never did. She *insisted* on always doing this stupid thing where she'd poke the inside of her cheek with my dick. I guess this was supposed to be a visual thing but it didn't do anything for me and she refused to stop doing it. It was like she was more interested in posing with my dick for some nonexistent camera than actually getting me off."

—*Rob, 26*

12. "Here's what happened:

Me: 'Spit on it more.'
Her: 'I don't like when there's a lot of spit everywhere.'
Me: 'It will make it wetter though.'
Her: 'Yeah, but it's gross."

She then proceeded to slowly tear the skin off my dick for five minutes until I asked her to stop."

—*Karl, 24*

13. "Um, if you can't deep throat then don't force yourself to try. Had one girl do this and it clearly hurt her throat terribly. It hurt my dick terribly too but she wouldn't stop trying aaaaand eventually she vomited on me. What a great evening that turned out to be."

—*Joey, 25*

14. "My main complaint is women with heavy hands who don't seem to know how hard or light they're squeezing and who seem completely unaware that they have back teeth. Seriously, think about it, what if I just alternated gnawing your nipples and sucking them while slapping your tits? Would that be an experience you'd be excited to have?"

—*Alvin, 28*

15. "Just swallow, I almost don't care what else you do. Just do that and I'll be happy. Sorry, I don't have a lot else to add."

—*Dirk, 20*

16. "The thing most likely to make a blowjob mediocre and forgettable or even unpleasant is the notion that some women have that there's no wrong way to give a blowjob and that guys are just so lucky to receive them. I've received blowjobs from dozens of women. The only ones I remember were where the lady cared about whether or not it felt good."

—*Nicholas, 30*

17. "Blowjobs are where you figure out whether or not you have a selfish lover. If she doesn't like to give them because of the taste then you've probably got a dead fish on your hands. I figure there's a lot of reasons not to like giving blowjobs but after going down on my fair share of women just days removed from their menses, without complaint I might add, 'I don't like the taste of your very clean dick' becomes a weak excuse."

—*Rick, 29*

18. "Don't use your teeth. Do incorporate your hand or hands. Do get it wet. Don't stop a lot. Most girls have this stuff all figured out but it seems like a lot of those that don't simply do not care to do it right."

—*Jason, 27*

12

Dear Gay Dude: My Girlfriend Won't S My D!

Ryan O'Connell

Dear Gay Dude,

I've been with this girl for the last few months and she's pretty awesome. She doesn't take any shit, she makes me laugh and she has an amazing body. Our sex life is pretty phenomenal too except for one major detail. She NEVER gives me head. One night, she grazed the tip with her tongue, but then quickly got out of there. What's the issue? Is my dick offensive? How do I suggest she suck my dick without coming off like a creepy asshole?

-Blowjobless

Dear Blowjobless,

As a gay man, I'm privy to all sorts of information about straight girls. Remember, they come to me to talk about *your* dick and any other sex issues, and here's what I've learned throughout the years: Girls don't really like to give blowjobs. I mean some of them do and if you happen to find one of those girls, you hold on to her tight, okay? In general though, straight girls view blowjobs as something you only do on a special occasion. Perhaps if they had a dick and knew what it felt like to have a mouth on it, they would be like gay men and want to give them all the time. But, alas, they don't so it's merely a job to them, which you can't blame them for. Giving a BJ is an exhausting process and I suggest you try doing it before you judge a girl for abstaining.

But here's how to increase your odds. First, do you go down on your girlfriend? If not, you don't need a Nancy Drew to figure out why she's dissing your dick. You need to give her private parts some one-on-one Sade time too. Otherwise, why the hell should she do the same for you? I've spoken to a lot of girls with vagina shame who give their boyfriends head without getting anything in return. And they're like, "I don't like it when he does it. It's gross. He doesn't need to do it. I don't want him to!" This defense is so sad. *Of course* you like getting eaten out. There's no way you don't. Seriously, it's just not possible. You just don't think you like it because A) you have some deep-seeded issues with your lady parts. Maybe you think it's ugly or smells weird. To which I say, what do you think a penis is? A work of art? Our genitalia always has the potential to look terrifying, but we get over it because we care more about someone touching it and making us feel good. Or B) your boyfriend doesn't know how to eat you out. He tries with gusto, but he fails miserably and you just can't deal with it so you tell him you don't like it.

Try eating your GF out and if she's like, "OMG NO!" you

have to be like, "I love you and your vagina. Just sit back and relax!" and do the damn thing. Afterwards, she'll be grateful and most likely give you head. In the odd event she's not reciprocating, just ask her flat out if she can give you a blowjob. I know it's not ideal, but communication is key. Tell her what's up (besides your dick) and be like, "It would be really great if you could do this for me." If she still takes a pass, she's a selfish lover and so not worth it.

God, I really hope this advice gets you a great blowjob. Good luck!

Love,

Gay Dude

13

Inner Monologue Of Someone Getting A Blowjob

Ryan O'Connell

Are they going to go down on me? God, I hope so. Blowjobs are so cool. Oh, look at that, they're kissing my stomach. I guess I better suck in a little bit. Now they're kissing around my hips and are almost to my penis. Oh my god, they're like two kisses away from landing on my actual penis. Here they go, getting closer and closer. Closer. CLOSER. And… wait, where is their mouth going? Come back! Did they just do a drive-by? Shit. Okay, I guess I have to wait before they decide to make their way back down there again. It's like Cher says in *Clueless* when they go to that party in the Valley: "Let's do a lap around the area before we commit to a location." The same goes for giving head.

I'm waiting…

Still waiting.

Jesus, they're giving my clavicle head before they even touch my penis.

Okay, now I think they're going in.

Oh, oh! And we have contact! A mouth is definitely on my penis. Thank god, No backing out now! You've signed the blowjob contract with your tongue and now you're stuck with my dick! Ha ha! (P.S. I love you.)

Hmm.

Well, this is weird. I don't feel anything.

I'm looking down and I can clearly see that they're doing things to my penis but why isn't it translating? My brain is not registering this blowjob. It's #NotClearOn me getting head right now.

Oh god, now I know why. They're not using their hands! They're treating my dick with the utmost care when really all it needs is to get beat up a bit. Penises aren't fragile, you know! They're designed to survive wars! Have you ever seen a guy jack off before? They're basically just murdering their penis until cum comes out of it. That's what it is, a murder, and honey when you're giving me head, I WANT YOU TO KILL MY DICK. I want it to be barely breathing by Duncan Sheik. Smack it around a little bit, give it a black eye. Don't be shy, just give it a try!

Okay, now they're using their hands. Oh, this feels damn good. I especially like it when they go down on my dick and then break for air, using their fresh saliva as lubrication to jack me off. That moment almost brings me to cum town but I resist blowing my load because I want the BJ to last longer. Granted, I don't want it to last *too* long. That would be rude. Giving a blowjob can be a nightmare, I know from personal experience, so I empathize. You gotta be respectful of the work that goes into it and make sure you cum under a certain time limit. If you're nervous about being able to do so, be a cheerleader for your own penis by screaming, "You can do it, dick! I believe in you! Cum, cum, cum!"

Shit, now that I think about it, I think I might be taking too long to cum. I see them working so hard down there. They're sweating and making obligatory moaning noises. I know that they must be thinking, "Jesus, hurry the fuck up and cum so we can order Thai food and watch a Pay-Per-View movie." They hate this. They're exhausted. I'm a failure for not cumming in an appropriate amount of time!

Uh-oh, I'm starting to feel anxiety. This isn't good. Anxiety is the silent killer of any sexual experience. It ruins everything. I just feel so bad that they're down there working their ass off and I'm just laying back and doing nothing. I should be contributing somehow. After all, this is a recession! You got to pull your own weight. Their job is to suck my dick and my job is to cum, and so far I'm not holding up on my end of things.

Okay, now my anxiety about cumming is preventing me from actually cumming. I'm so frustrated. I'd tell my brain to go suck my dick but...

Okay, I know what I'm going to do. I'm going to go to my favorite fantasy in my brain to get myself back on track. La la la, dee, dee, dee. Okay, I'm there. Things feel good. Now I'm inching towards semen. I can sense it.

Oh my god, wait, I think I'm almost there. I better scream it! There. I screamed it.

Wait, false alarm. Shit. "JK!" I squeak.

OK, now I'm almost there for real. My leg is even doing that weird leg cramp thing it does before I climax. It's sort of painful actually.

Oh my god oh my god oh my god semen is traveling through me and about to land somewhere that's not inside my body yes yes yes yes!

My toes curl up, my head goes back, and boom, we're having a baby! Just kidding. I just came in your hair. God, that felt good.

Wait, what are you doing? Are you still jacking me off after I cum? Please don't. My dick is very sensitive right now and touching it is causing my body to twitch. I'm seriously twitching! Hands off my penis! It's in a weird place right now.

Oh, thank god, they saw my leg twitching and took that as a cue to stop. Now we're just lying there exhausted. I feel like I ran a marathon, even though I didn't even move. That was great. I'm so proud of both of us for that successful blowjob. We're two sexually healthy human beings. We've been validated.

Now let's order some Thai.

14

10 People Share Their Hilarious First Blowjob Stories

Tatiana Pérez

1. "It was my sophomore year of high school and I was on vacation with my family in Cancun. All my friends had gotten head already and I was really anxious and extremely wasted, so I panicked and solicited a questionably very old street-walker. The next morning, I realized she'd stolen the family vacation camera from my back pocket. Worst part, though? I was so hammered and nervous that I didn't even bust. She left me pants down in the middle of the alley where she'd started the job. No camera, no cum. Brutal."

—Imran, 22

2. "We were both 16, and he was my boyfriend at the time. My more experienced friends had given me a slew of tips—cover your teeth, incorporate your hands, look up at him while you do it. I was well-studied. The moment it started happening, though, all those hours of planning and practicing on bananas (yes, I *actually* practiced on bananas… and the occasional cucumber) went right out the window. I had no idea what the *fuck* I was doing. Then, my boyfriend started bleeding. Like, his penis literally started to *bleed* because I'd scratched some skin off with my teeth. Brilliant. We stayed together for a while after that and remain really good friends. He's uncircumcised and I'm Jewish, so to this day, we refer to that night as his bris."

—*Sami, 21*

3. "The first one wasn't that exhilarating. It was before I came out, and it was in a laundry room. I was super embarrassed because I hadn't shaved and I thought this girl was gonna think I was dirty. Then after I came out she told everyone she knew I was gay because I didn't have a boner when she blew me. But I was rocking a half-chub, and she fucking knows it."

—*Zach, 24*

4. "When I was in third grade, my older sister told me what a blowjob was. I was fascinated… a penis in your mouth? And you… suck on it? Like candy? Bizarre. She told me that people 'normally' give/receive head by 15, so naturally, I was determined to have my debut before then. I was an aggressive kid. Skip to five years later, and it's the eve of my 15th birthday. I still hadn't given one, but I wasn't giving up. I IM-ed this boy from the grade above who had eyes for me and was a notorious slut. I told him to meet me the next morning at the one unisex bathroom at our school, minutes before my bio final. I got to work, and I killed it. He came in like two minutes, max. I wiped my mouth, stood up, said 'thank you,' and ran to my exam. When I got there, my teacher noted that I had some white stuff on my lip. You guessed it! Jizz. Jizz on my lip for my

100-year-old bio teacher to see. To this day, whenever I finish giving head, I imagine my old ass teacher giving me that mortifying *heads up* (ha)."

—*Adrienne, 21*

5. "I got my first blowjob when I was 17 in the middle of our family living room at 6 a.m. This incredibly sexy girl had slept over at my house and she was trying to slip out early, so I walked her to the door. Then, right by our piano, she turned to me, put her hand on my dick, and slipped my boxers off. She sat on the piano stool and proceeded to suck. I was about to come when I felt something wet on my ass. It was my dog's tongue. She'd been sitting right behind me for who knows how long, innocently watching this girl go down on me while she licked my butt. Something about it was so horrifying—Roxy, the dog I've had since I was a baby, weirdly involved in my first BJ—that I immediately went soft. Roxy's never looked at me the same, I swear."

—*Marc, 20*

6. "I was 16 and I was a counselor in training at my camp. There was this guy I'd been hooking up with all summer, and it was the kind of thing where, like, we both knew it was *the night.* We went to the basement of this party cabin the counselors had rented for us, very awkwardly silent, and entered this weird room where everything was orange. Like… everything. That's where it happened. I remember fixating on this particularly orange lava lamp while I grew genuinely afraid that I was gonna bite his dick off and/or that saliva might never return to my mouth because it felt so excruciatingly dry.

Then my friend started pounding on the door. I was so rattled that I popped up and shattered the lava lamp. I don't remember if he finished or not."

—Kendall, 19

7. "It was the summer after my freshman year of high school. I was 15 and she was 17, so as you can imagine, I was beyond pumped to have this hot, older girl christen my penis. My house was on a lake and we had one of those long piers that extended out into the water, and that's where it went down—at the very edge of the pier. Hot, right? Right. Very hot. She was incredible. The finale was so intense that it knocked me of my feet… literally. As in, I came so forcefully that I fell into the lake, shorts around my ankles."

—Marcel, 20

8. "The first time I gave head was also the first time I kissed a guy. He was 24 and I was 18, but I lied and told him I was 21. I'd been going down on him for what felt like hours when I felt my phone buzzing in my pocket. I obviously didn't plan on picking up, but somehow, my ass answered for me. All of the sudden, I heard my mom screaming into the phone. 'Nick??? NICK, WHERE ARE YOU?!' It was 3 a.m. and I hadn't called or texted to say I'd be home late, which was really rare for me. But I was distracted, you know, by the blowjob/my first gay sex experience. Now I had to pick up. The guy listened, clearly horrified, as I anxiously explained to my mother that I'd be home in no time. When I hung up, he just quietly goes, '21, huh?' I was mortified. I literally said nothing as I gathered my things and fled the scene."

—Nick, 22

9. "All throughout high school, I took a moral stance against blowjobs. I wasn't a prude or anything… actually, I lost my virginity at 15, which I feel is pretty young. For whatever reason, though, I found them degrading, and I just had zero interest in shoving a hairy, ugly penis down my throat. Fast forward to my freshman year in college, and my tune had totally changed. I was hooking up with this devilishly hot guy one night and decided that it was now or never. Of course, we were both totally trashed. So trashed that, immediately after he came, the guy vomited right on his floor… and then I vomited. Everywhere. Literally… everywhere. Like, his room was covered in puke. That was the first and last blowjob I ever gave."

—*Raquel, 23*

10. "I was in 8th grade and my 'girlfriend' (girl who'd been letting me kiss her for the past month or so) had made the very exiting promise of giving me my first blowjob one weekend my parents were gonna be away. I really set the mood—candles and shit, the whole thing. She'd yet to touch my penis—no girl had. I was so hyped. She came over and we started making out immediately. Just the thought of what was coming had gotten me harder than I'd ever been. Like… very, very hard. So hard that, when I felt her hands inching toward my dick, I came. On the spot, just like that. We were both extremely rattled. She stopped texting back, and I didn't end up getting a BJ until a year later, when the exact same thing *almost* happened."

—*Jorge, 21*

15

How To Give A (Good) Blowjob

Jillian Paulson

Never give the same blowjob twice. That's boring. You don't like to be fucked the same way every single time, do you? No, you don't. So return the favor.

Don't go right into sucking dick. Make him wait a little bit. Tease him a little. Don't just slide down and clamp your mouth right on his cock. If he's lying down, run your body up and down his chest. Brush your tits against his skin. Kiss his neck while you run your hand towards his dick. Lightly scratch his thighs. Trace a path down his body with your lips very gently till he shivers. YOU decide when to take it in your mouth, not him. I like to take just the head in my mouth and lick its underside gently a few times before I start working.

Take your goddamn time! Once you have it in your mouth, don't go from licking to sucking to hardcore bobbing in under five minutes. That's what you did in high school and you have no business doing that shit now.

A good blowjob is like a slow-cooker. The longer you let it

cook, the better it is. He'll totally fall apart in your hands. (Or your mouth, I suppose.)

Use your hands. Always, always, always use your hands. You can finger yourself with one hand so you're getting something out of this experience, but the power of a hand and your mouth is unparalleled. Lube your hand up with that good, slimy spit in the back of your throat and use it as an extension of your mouth. Not too tight, but not gentle either. Keep a firm grip on that dick. I like to alternate using my whole hand and just a few fingers. A popular trick I discovered is making a ring shape with my thumb and two fingers and sliding that over the head and down like it's attached to my mouth. Tight feels good. Remember that.

Act like you like it. You should be enjoying it anyway; if you need encouragement, just remember how much power you have over him in this moment. He is at your mercy. This is not a chore. Giving is fun. Enjoy it. Moan a little. That stupid "Cosmo" tip about humming the Star-Spangled Banner is true; men really like a little vibration. But don't hum the national anthem, OK? He's not gonna enjoy it as much if you make it feel like a chore.

Give him a show. He's gonna be watching you while you're down there, so look up at him and hold his gaze for a few moments while you take his dick in your mouth. They go CRAZY for that shit. They love watching it slide in and out of your mouth or watching your tongue flick away as you lick. Talk dirty—this is a good tip if you need a minute to breathe normally. Tell him you love sucking his big cock. ("Big cock" seems to be magic words for dudes.)

Get creative. Take your panties off and wrap them around the base of his dick. Don't be boring. Take your time—you don't like short-ass head sessions, and neither does he. Stop for a minute and let him watch you touch your nipples or play with yourself.

Watch and listen to him for cues to figure out what he likes. Alternate between slow, teasing licks and quick, tight sucking movements in and out of your mouth to build up the tension. Once he's getting close, cup his balls in one hand as you suck—they LOVE that. (Side note: Don't ignore the balls. Lick 'em. Suck 'em. Dudes like it and balls get wrongly ignored in Blowjob Land. I'm a fan of balls. I give them their due attention.)

And don't fucking spit out the cum, OK? Suck it down. Get excited about it. You did it, didn't you? You are the catalyst for this cum situation! Be proud of yourself.

16

What I Love (And Hate) About Blowjobs

Jillian Paulson

Sometimes when I have him in my mouth I look up and I think, "I could do anything to you right now."

They look so stupid when you're blowing them. They're all blissed out with their eyes rolling all around in their head. Or you're making eye contact with them as you blow them because that's what the magazines tell you to do. I always get my hair in my eyes so it's probably less sexy, but they don't seem to notice cause I'm working my magic on their dick.

Just blink every once in awhile, buddy, you're scaring me.

The worst ones put their hands all in your hair and fuck it up. The ultimate worst push your head down, but I don't fuck with those dudes anymore. If you wanna try that, you're gonna get a little more teeth on your precious thin-skinned dick than you bargained for.

The good ones react just the way you want them to: panting, moaning, writhing around. They aren't thinking that at any minute you could bite down, or yank too hard on their balls.

You wouldn't anyway, would you? No, you just think about it sometimes. But I always thought that if I were gonna kill a man I would do it while giving him head. They'll tell you anything you want if you've got your lips around their pride and joy. You can get whatever you want from them: oh baby, give me a diamond, give me a treat, give me give me give me. And they'll say they will, because their brain is shut off and all they can feel are those nerve endings humming and that vacuuming motion of your mouth. If you hold them to those promises, well, that's up to you.

But don't get me wrong, I really truly do love giving a good blowjob, cause nothing's better than when you finish and the dude doesn't even remember his own name. You get a mouthful of frothy, salty cum as your reward. I've done so many for various boyfriends and random guys that I don't have to focus as hard anymore. It's going through the motions for most of them.

A blowjob is gonna make any man happy—period. They love that shit. I'm good at them; they all tell me in breathless tones how good I am when I suck down their cum after making them bust like a freight train.

It's fun to slide down their body and then hear them gasp when you slide that whole length right down your damn throat. The further you can slide it, the better the spit for lube. Then when you get bored with routine licking and sucking, you add a hand or two and they really flip shit. My favorite thing to do is make a fist at the tip and then slip my tongue through it really slowly, squeezing just a little as I slide his dick through said fist. He hits the roof every time.

Once you really get going and you cough up a little spit from your throat, you can get as many inches as you want down your throat. Little by little, girl, and then you can conquer it.

17

13 Women Describe What They Love Most About Going Down On Their Boyfriends

Mélanie Berliet

1. "Whenever I give my boyfriend a blowjob, I amuse myself by experimenting with different ways to think about his dick. Like, I'll pretend it's a harmonica one minute, and then I'll segue into picturing it as a lollipop or a Popsicle. I love using my imagination to change things up and keep things interesting for both of us."

—*Missy, 23*

2. "I'm a feminist, but I'm not afraid to say that I feel validated when I make my man ejaculate. It helps that my boyfriend's semen tastes pretty good. But I don't always swallow. Sometimes I tell him to spray it all over my face for effect."

—*Kendall, 20*

3. "Sucking dick isn't exactly a treat, but it's not unpleasant, either. It's like sitting through a beautiful foreign film when you're not exactly in the mood to read subtitles. There's a definite payoff, but you have to put some work into it. What I like about giving head is that feeling of accomplishment I get from it. "

—*Ramona, 32*

4. "Personally, I love ball play. Some girls think balls are gross or whatever, but only because they aren't used to them. Once you know what you're dealing with, testicles are a really useful pleasure enhancing tool. I'm pretty sure I won my boyfriend over with my ball massaging talents alone."

—*Lyla, 26*

5. "My boyfriend is *really* well endowed, which is great during sex but not when I'm giving him head. At first it was really upsetting, actually. I felt like a failure because I couldn't fit that much of him in my mouth. But the situation forced me to get creative—to figure out how to use my hands and mouth in different ways. I approach the blowie like the art form it is these days. It's challenging but satisfying, especially when he finally comes."

—*Anne Marie, 28*

6. "A lot of women resent it when a man shoves their head down with his hand, but I honestly love the hand-on-head thing. In my relationship, at least, it's not about submission or dominance. It's about rhythm. If I pay attention to the gentle pressure my boyfriend puts on my head, I know exactly how to pace myself and it makes me feel connected to him."

—*Kate, 29*

7. "I'm dating a guy who squirms *a lot* during oral and I love watching his hips wriggle and shift. Every pelvic movement confirms that I'm doing something right."

—*Victoria, 21*

8. "The best part of a good fellatio session is getting something in return. Not a sexual favor, but a present or something else I want on any particular day, like a double date with a couple my boyfriend doesn't really like. I'm definitely not above giving a blowjob with a distinct purpose in mind."

—*Terry, 35*

9. "My current partner's uncircumcised. I'd never seen foreskin up close until we started dating, and I was instantly fascinated by it. I'm convinced he feels more pleasure when I play with it and I love using that to my advantage when I'm giving him a BJ."

—*Olivia, 23*

10. "You know the rim of a penis, where the shaft meets the head? I recently learned that part has its own name: the corona. I worship my boyfriend's corona because tonguing it drives him crazy. That's easily the best part about going down on him."

—*Finn, 25*

11. "I'm guessing I'm not alone in feeling like the absolute best part about giving any guy head is how nicely he treats you immediately afterwards. From my experience, they're especially grateful if it's a wake-and-suck situation, which I tend to reserve for special occasions like birthdays and anniversaries."

—Daria, 31

12. "Whatever makes the 'job' aspect easiest is what I'm into. So whatever gets him off fastest. Thing is, you can't assume it's always the same thing. Could be a little ball rubbing one afternoon and some gentle taint tickling the next."

—Brooke, 27

13. "My boyfriend's dick is below average in size—not too small that it's a problem during sex, but small enough that blowing him is a piece of fucking delicious cake. I feel like a total pro when I give him head, and that's a good feeling to have. There's so much hype about big dicks but I'm a fan of the just right cock hanging between my boyfriend's legs."

—Nicolette, 31

18

If You Want A Blowjob, Wash Your Damn Dicks

Madison Moore

This is an urgent message to ya'll men. This boy told me to tell ya'll, ya'll need to wash under ya'll damn nuts, and all around ya'll damn nuts. Even if you do not get penetrated and have anal seks, then you still have an obligation to lift yo' nut sack UP and go all underneath the crack, around the back of ya'll nuts. And then all around the dick, too. They say the dick be stankin, especially if you got that foreskin around ya'll dick. They said ya'll don't be pulling that dick back to get all that grease and backed up funk and shit caked all around ya'll dick!

Guys love getting head but not everybody likes doing it. Some say its too subservient, others just don't like it. But have you ever gone down on a guy and as soon as you reached the nether region all you got was a big whiff of dirty dick funk? SERIOUSLY right now? There is no excuse for having a funky dick! A person is about to put their mouth on your penis and their face in your pubes for 5 to 45 minutes. Be hospitable!

Treat them to a comfy, pleasant experience. I've never been confronted with dirty dick syndrome myself but apparently it's enough of a thing that Miss Ask Alexyss herself had to make a Youtube video reminding guys everywhere to wash their damn dicks. And when Ask Alexyss has to come for you, oh you know it's bad.

Consider yourselves warned, blowjob seekers!

19

13 Men On The One Thing They Wish All Women Knew About Giving Head

Tatiana Pérez

1. "It's like anything else with sex—I'm more into it if she's more into it."

—Amar, 21

2. "If you can use your mouth to create a vacuum force equal to that of a Dyson while simultaneously keeping it wetter than a tsunami in Bikini Bottom, you will definitely be able to pleasure any man."

—Jackson, 23

3. "Don't be afraid to yank on it."

—Oscar, 25

4. "I feel like women think they've gotta go ham on my dick to make me cum. Not the case. I like a slow burn."

—*Luis, 22*

5. "Less hands, more mouth. Always."

—*Kyle, 24*

6. "Don't act like you're in a porno. Contrary to what you've seen, choking and gagging is not very hot. In fact, it's often somewhat disturbing."

—*Wolfgang, 23*

7. "Take off your damn rings."

—*Ray, 19*

8. "Give my balls some love. It's not a blowjob till the whole crew is involved."

—*Mac, 21*

9. "Swallowing never hurts."

—*Howe, 23*

10. "My girlfriend likes to put my hands on the back of her head when she's going down on me. I fucking love that."

—*Lucas, 25*

11. "I don't wanna say 'please let me face-fuck you,' but I do love a woman who's down for me to move my hips."

—*Olin, 22*

12. "Patience is a major key. If I'm taking a while to come, it doesn't mean you're doing a bad job at all. It generally takes longer than sex."

—*Winston, 20*

13. "Eye contact is huge. Doesn't seem that easy, but if you can pull it off, bravo."

—*Nico, 27*

20

3 Spectacular Steps To An Unbeatable Blowjob

Sofia Green

Step I

Begin by making out with him and kind of leaning your thigh between his legs. Eventually transition to pushing him into a sitting position where you are on your knees between his thighs. Unbutton just the top of your shirt. Do not undo your bra, as you will need the push-up factor later. Take off his belt with one hand in a nimble, swift, bordering-on-violent way. Maintain eye contact and facial proximity during your destruction of his belt. He should be as hard as an Organic Chemistry final after this move. Lean his face forward so that you're still making out with him but your cleavage is basically hugging his dick. Move your torso in a slow up-and-down motion. If you're feeling particularly manipulative and/or sadistic, abruptly stop and suddenly realize that you're late for something; if you're in a public place, act like you heard someone coming. Abandon effort. He will be devastated, but chalk it up to inopportune timing.

Step II

When he's had ample time to fantasize about what the inside of your throat feels like, briefly repeat Step I at a later date. After considerable cleavage stimulation, grab the base of his dick firmly and put your mouth on the tip. Roll your tongue on the tip's underside. Don't go too overboard on this move, because that is both a little weird and specific. Then start accumulating spit in your mouth and put your lips in a kiss/duck face position and DISCREETLY let that saliva sort of leak out as you slide your duck face up and down the shaft. This is a strange-looking but necessary step, so make your face parallel with his body so that he can't see the tomfoolery going on with your mouth right now. Move your hand in tandem with this motion and when your lips get to the bottom of the shaft, cup his balls with your hand so they don't feel left out. By then his dick should be completely lubricated.

WARNING: By skipping this crucial step you will get dry mouth and he will get dry dick and no one is happy and everything is dry.

Step III

Congratulations! You made it to the finale.

You're wondering: "Why the fuck is this so long and instructional?" Because I'm very detail-oriented and also a little drunk right now. So…

Wrap upper lips over top row of teeth like you are imitating a toothless old person. Stick out tongue flatly so it shields bottom teeth. Again, hide your face with your hair or something because you've never looked more ridiculous than you do right now. Begin to bob up and down on his dick slowly at first. This part should not take long but if it does, god bless your soul.

If you get tired, give your neck a break and go back to the beginning of Step II while looking coyly into his eyes as if you are enjoying it. If you get really tired, take an extended break by whispering into his ear how wet this makes you and guide his hand to prove it. This provides a neck break and also stimulation for you—clearly a win-win. Eventually go back to the finale and try not to drag your feet about it, as it will be over soon and if it isn't, then he should be kind enough to throw in the towel.

Once his legs get sort of twitchy or he verbally says he's cumming or moans or whatever cue, then comes the most important part. While bobbing your head, pause when the tip is at the farthest back part of your throat and make sure he cums way at the back of your throat. This is so it just sort of falls down there and no swallowing or gargling or sampling of the baby batter actually occurs. Let gravity swallow it for you. Don't spit it out or be awkward about it, because that is messy and just ruins the illusion after all of that neck straining.

If you want to get a little dirtier, let just one drop come out of the side of your mouth and wipe it away with one finger and then lick that finger while maintaining eye contact. This is obviously reserved for guys you actually respect or have feelings for, because if you do this with a rando they will tell all their friends you may be a porn star. If you're feeling especially freaky and don't mind messes, pull it out before he cums and allow the explosion to happen on your cleavage. For the love of god, be careful where you pull this absurd move because no one wants to explain to—hypothetically, of course—their boss after lunch hour why there are interesting stains on your shirt.

Be warned. This formula yields strong results. It was developed over the years through extensive fieldwork and creates frightening amounts of commitment from the recipient. It's dangerous knowledge and when applied wisely, you can hold the keys to the world. I suspect Monica Lewinsky used this very same formula. One day I hope I get the chance to ask her.

Now get out there and suck some dick!

21

The Big Gulp: 10 People On The First Time They Swallowed

Kat George

1. "The first time I swallowed I ran away from my boyfriend, spit it out in the sink, and took a swig chocolate syrup. He was a Christian. He wanted me to put the syrup on his dick. I wouldn't. He currently lives in Denver with his boyfriend."

—*Lia, 25*

2. "Swallowing is funny because it seems like there is such a premium on it, versus "spitting" which takes more skill anyways. The first time I swallowed I didn't even know what I was doing, it just happened. Like, suddenly there was this rush of salty liquid in my mouth, no warning. It was cool, I think. It was nice that there was a very concrete end point because otherwise I would have had no idea when to be done, at that point."

—*Christine, 28*

3. "Ok so I can't remember the FIRST time I swallowed. but O can remember a series of times. honestly at this point I don't even remember spitting ever. I think for me swallowing and sucking dick go hand in hand. spitting always seemed too messy, too much of a—the first words that came to mind were dick/pussy, I don't know what that says about me BUT—seemed like too much of a dick move / a pussy move. i remember it being so fucking disgusting the first several times. Hell, it's even kind of gross now. I'm madly in love with my boyfriend and I still kind of gag a bit at the end of a BJ. For me that's the only option. The idea of spoiling the moment to run to the sink and spit? That doesn't appeal to me. And nothing turns me on more than when I'm told how good i taste, so then I would assume to reason that a man feels the same. I think if I were a dude and a girl was always spitting out my splooge, my feelings would be hurt. Really, I'm just protecting everyone's feelings. that's what's going on here."

—*Celeste, 27*

4. "It was with my first boyfriend, who was emotionally abusive and extremely selfish. The first time I swallowed was not my choice and I had no warning. He wouldn't kiss me afterwards and shortly asked me to leave."

—*Alex, 21*

5. "The first time I swallowed jizz I threw it up 5 minutes later. It was disgusting. It was so horrible, I was like yeah man I can do this, I can totally swallow jizz. I was like 19, and it was a huge load too and I was like OH OK THEN and then it tasted so wrong, like off milk mixed with ball sweat and so I swallowed it… then I tried to remain suave and sexy… then my stomach was churning and I threw up gluggy hot semen and it was the most disgusting feeling rising up from my throat into my mouth."

—Courtney, 25

6. "I had been going out with this guy for about a month and a half. I was on my period and really didn't want to get his sheets messy but he kept saying he didn't mind and that it was fine with him. But since we were still pretty new, I really wanted to wait before we got into the period sex thing so I decided to go down on him instead. While I was blowing him, he kept saying how good it was and that he was close—you know, the usual pep talk. So I was really into it and when he told me he was about to come I just kept going and let him come in my mouth. At that moment, spitting it out didn't seem like an option so I went ahead and swallowed it. The weird thing is, couple of seconds after I had swallowed, he looked up and asked me if I swallowed it and I got nervous and said "yeah, some of it". His response to that was "ohh okay, cuz we haven't been going out for that long so I don't think we're there yet." We went out for another month after that but I never swallowed his again."

—Amy, 23

7. "The first time I ever did it was with my first semi serious boyfriend (I lost my virginity to him the night of my year 10 formal. How original). Anyways a few months before that he wanted me to give him head and I had only done it once before with one of my friends older brothers who told me after I had let him cum all over himself that in order to give great head you should swallow. So I took his advice and when my boyfriend said he was going to cum I said ok with a mouthful of cock. He said it was the best head he ever had so I was convinced that swallowing really was the key and I have done it every time since. Obviously I don't still believe it is all about the swallow but it definitely helps Plus it always makes me feel superior to girls who refuse to."

—*Ashleigh, 26*

8. "Nathan and I had planned to go to his student accommodation for a quick smoke then take the bus into town for a drink; a first date as it were. Three hefty joints later and the sound of Primal Scream ringing in my ear the sexual tension had grown unbearable between us; to the point where we had silences simply looking at each other with raised eyebrows waiting for something to happen. The atmosphere was not even stifled by the awful lighting and interiors which looked fresh out of One Flew Over the Cuckoos Nest. Finally he made the first move and my teenage instinct went into overdrive and I jumped on him, grinding him rigorously and tugging at his belt. One thing led to another and all of a sudden he was fucking my (almost) virgin mouth. I'd like to think I knew what I was doing; I just gave it dedication and effort which was increasingly difficult in my stoned state with my mouth becoming more and more dry, the viscosity of my saliva becoming more like treacle (sorry for the graphic imagery, I just don't know how else to put it) but heck! I went for it, and after about 3 minutes of cock-sucking dedication his body tensed and a jet of salty come exploded into my mouth. Ugh, do I swallow it? Is there anywhere to spit? It's on my hands, uh no, it's on my dress too, oop and now it's in my hair... and some in my eye. THIS SHIT GET'S EVERY-WHERE. I thought I'd be kinky and lick it up though which really didn't help my dry mouth. The fact that I walked home that evening with dried jizz on my nylon black dress just showed how much I didn't give a fuck. When I told Nathan he just laughed and stroked his beard. Moral of the story; Giving blowjobs when high is CHALLENGING. Proceed with caution."

—Bryony, 19

9. "First time I swallowed was the first blowjob I ever gave. I wanted to impress and thought it would be hot. Well, tasted like ass. At the time I didn't know any better but I was seriously re-evaluating how "hot" I thought it was. That ex ate a lot of fast food and I later learned that was why it tasted so bad. Eat fruit! Once I "discovered" that trick future lovers got that and it got way better for me. Now, about 4 years later. I loooove it, it's incredibly hot."

—Geill, 22

10. "The first time I swallowed I was at a Westfield in the suburbs in the parking lot in an older guy's car. I was fourteen and he must have been at least thirty—I organized the meeting on gaydar. Then I got out. And I got a Boost Juice. And found my parents. True story."

—Craig, 22

22

True Story: I Puked On My Crushes' Dick

Anonymous

We have to throwback to '03 where all good stories start; junior high. I went to a private school that always invited a similar private school to all their school dances. Being the "before my time kind of girl," I asked this cute boy to dance. He accepted my offer; we probably danced to "Hero" by Enrique Iglesias, exchanged names. For the purposes of this story let's call him Sebastian and then we parted ways. Apparently he could turn up those moves because I had a major crush on this dude for a solid month, and then forgot he existed.

Ten years later, my ex boyfriend of two and a half years recently dumped my ass for another girl and I was on a slut spree. I had stayed in my hometown for my entire undergraduate degree; I was on the brink of graduating and getting the fuck out of there. I signed up for an intensive program in Montreal for the summer and I decided that I was going to figure out a way to stay there. I was at the bar for my friends' birthday, and as I was standing waiting for my drink I saw this hot guy standing next to me that looked very familiar. This guy and I simultaneously approached each other and started talking. I asked him what his name was and he said Sebastian. Turns out he was fully my junior high crush and I was pretty drunk so I blurted that out. He obviously did not remember me. We talked a bit and he said he came back home after finishing his degree and was in the process of looking for a job in Montreal. He asked me to dance, we popped a molly, and he twirled me around the dance floor.

We went outside for a smoke and he asked if I wanted to get out of there and go to his friends place. When people usually mention going to a friends place at one thirty in the morning on a Saturday night, one would assume it's filled with people who are partying. Apparently not. We arrive at his friends' house in the middle of suburbia only to be greeted by his friend and his entire family, including their dog. I was flying and throwing back some wine in order to not look rude. I sat on their couch and talked to his friends' Mom for an hour.

By three in the morning his parents were ready for bed. Sebastian, his friend and I went downstairs to their basement, his friend started to watch TV and Sebastian was ready to get the real party started in the next room. I asked if he had a condom and he said no, and neither did his friend; I was not having any of that. He decided that we should go back to his place, despite apparently having a pretty strict household. We call a cab, say bye to his friend and we were on our way. We stopped on our way so Sebastian could take out money to pay the cab driver and he asked if I needed anything. I told him I would like a pack of gum because my jaw was a clenching mess. He comes back to the cab with five different flavors of gum. We get back to his house, fuck, talk about books, Montreal and then fall asleep. Sebastian wakes me up, tells me it would be a good time for me to leave, as his Mom is out for a morning stroll. He grabs me a cab, paid for the cab, claims he'll text me on Tuesday and sends me on my way. Tuesdays comes, no text, I figured it was just a one-night stand.

During my last week of exams in April, I was checking my old Hotmail account and I saw there was an email from the alumni office of my high school. I opened it, it's from some weird name, who says he is an old friend of mine inquiring how to contact me. Who the fuck is this. I send back some sassy reply, thinking it's some dumb prank. A few hours later, I get a reply and it's Sebastian. He apparently got a new phone and had to get crafty to find me (my Facebook is unsearchable). I added him on Facebook and we discussed a time and a place to meet up. He said that he got a job in Montreal and was leaving at the end of the month. Due to his limited time, we would have to get together for drinks in a less than ideal "I'll bring a friend, you bring a friend situation." Drinks were going well, I mentioned that I booked my flight to Montreal and we should meet up while I'm there, he seemed down. Everyone's having a good time but both our friends were ready to call it a night.

We both knew what was up next; I didn't drive to the lounge, so we got in his car, which happened to be his parents' mini van and parked on a random residential street to hook up. Neither of us was in the position to have the other over. I was pretty tipsy and so was he. I had my period so I wasn't really down to have sex, since this was only our second time hooking up. I started giving him a blowjob. I was deep throating him to the extreme; he seemed to be really enjoying himself, he was thrusting his penis as I tried to go further down his shaft, the greedy kid just wanted more. He thrusted and pretty much tried to fuck my mouth, before I had time to react I projectile vomited on my seventh grade crushes' penis. Who seriously projectile vomits on their grade 7 crushes' penis, apparently I do! I instantly covered my mouth, died inside and said, "I need a fucking cigarette."

Probably, the most embarrassing moment of my life to date. He was not impressed by any means. Like seriously not impressed. He dropped me off at home; he said he had to volunteer at a hospital early the next morning, out of all the excuses to use! The next day I sent him a text apologizing, he replied and everything seemed cool. The following Thursday was my last two exams; of course they're on the same day, back to back. I was planning on going out after and getting wasted. Sebastian and I discussed meeting up sometime during the night, but it just didn't turn out. He invited me to his pre-drink, which was too far from where I was at the time. We ended up at different clubs and it just didn't work out. I left for vacation on the following Saturday and I figured he was on his way back to Montreal. We spoke a few times after that but nothing that substantial.

A month goes by, I was creeping Facebook and noticed that he deleted me off Facebook!! After an intensive creep session

I figured out he had a girlfriend the entire time! Obviously, I deleted his phone number and didn't bother texting him over the summer. I ended up figuring out a reason to stay in Montreal and still haven't given a blowjob since. Moral of the story, giving a blowjob is like someone giving you a gift, don't be too greedy or you'll end up with a lump of coal (or a pile of puke) in your lap!

23

Why I Love Sucking Dick

Anonymous

The last time I had sex I was blowing this guy and when I came up for air, to kiss him, he said, "Jesus, you are so good." What are you supposed to do when someone compliments you during sex? It didn't seem right to say, "Thank you, I have worked long and hard for these skills" so I just sort of smiled and kept going because I don't think he wanted me to stop.

I love sucking dick. I love the feeling of a dick at the back of my throat and I love opening his pants for the first time, not sure what's going to pop out. I love it when he kicks all the way back, manspreads, and I get to be on my knees worshiping his cock. I want him to caress my hair, stroke my face, toy with my ears and maybe gently guide me along. The best, though, is when I glance up at him and see that he is in such a state of ecstasy—eyes rolled back into his head, mouth slightly open. Look at what I can do to you.

What I love most about going down on my guy is that when it's as good for me as it is for him it really brings us closer together. Any good, mind-blowing sex should be about each of you reaching a peak.

Everyone who sucks penises thinks they're good at sucking penises. I have never heard anyone, gay or straight, say "I am such a terrible cocksucker." Have you? We might read articles online with useful tips or suggestions about how to give better dome, but nobody ever prefaces oral sex with, "I'll do it but I'm not very good" because that would kill the boner.

The secret to sucking excellent penis is not about cupping your hands or licking the head in a swirling motion or putting a mint in your mouth or eating an ice cube beforehand. That stuff's for amateurs. You just have to be dedicated. You have to really, really want to suck that dick. Lose yourself in the dick. This doesn't mean you need to eat the thing but you do have to be completely fascinated by it, the way it looks, the way it feels in your throat. You have to show that you can't get enough.

I have heard too many people say that sucking dick is degrading, that worshipping a dick or being on your knees in front of your man is dehumanizing. Dick sucking is power. You have the power to bring him to an orgasm, which he could do without you, sure, but he can't suck himself the way you can suck him. He needs you for that. He will remember how good you are and every time you have sex he'll be so eager to have you do his favorite thing. When you're out at dinner he'll look at you from across the table and will remember and when he flashes you a smile this is what he's thinking.

I suck dick because I want to. I really want to. So should you. But remember: it is not a race.

24

Inner Monologue Of A Person Giving A Blow Job

January Nelson

Giving an impromptu blow job pretty much grants automatic street cred to the dick sucker; and in that way, it's a total win-win. He's gonna get his dick sucked; I'm gonna get off on controlling his mind, body, and penis for the next ~20 minutes. There are no losers here.

[moments of unconscious sexual enjoyment]

I'm legitimately confused about how penises (penii?) taste so wonderful. I mean, it's just skin, but it's not salty or sweaty or... I don't know, it's like penii are immune to forces of nature that the rest of the body fall victim to. A penis doesn't taste like an armpit or a foot. A penis sets the bar for how flesh should taste. Or maybe it's just this particular penis I'm sucking. Maybe this one happens to be perfect.

[moments of unconscious sexual enjoyment]

What never ceases to amaze me about having a dick in my

mouth is how smooth the head is. Like, were you designed to be slobbered on, honey? Why are you so flawless and adorable? There is no part of the human anatomy that deserves the warmth and wetness of a mouth more than the tip of a penis. Even when I'm not in the mood, I see a hard penis all erect down there; and then the head, the icing on a shining penis-beacon of hope, and I'm like, "This beautiful specimen is proof that there's a god, hallelujah."

[moments of unconscious sexual enjoyment]

I could seriously fall asleep right now with just the tip in my mouth, but that probably wouldn't be much fun for the rest of the penis or for the person who's attached to it. Better move my way down a little. I guess I'll get some hand action in there, too.

[moments of unconscious sexual enjoyment]

God damn, this is a family affair. We've got hands, there's balls, the head, the shaft, my mouth… I mean, this takes a fuck-load of coordination and I'm not necessarily athletic but I'm gonna try my damnedest to see this thing through. I'm gonna suck that head, work that shaft, and mind those balls—I won-der if this guy knows sucking his dick is a freaking blue collar job. Seriously, I hope he's prepared to offer me workers' comp because if he doesn't come soon, I'm gonna have to take med-ical leave from penis-related activity.

[moments of belabored, but purposeful, sucking]

Should I suggest we fuck instead? Unless I get some pre-cum

to work with, my reservoir is about to dry up. There's only so much saliva in one mouth. Is it poor form to take a water break? I'm just gonna sit up for a second and jerk him off so I can replenish my natural resources.

[moments of hoping visual of breasts/ hand job is enough to suffice until strength has been regained]

All right, I'm back in the game. He's making affirming noises. Please, keep making those noises. I'm Tinker Bell and your moaning is the applause I need to keep me alive. Seriously, keep clapping or I will die down here.

[moments of summoning every ounce of moisture from mouth onto penis]

OK. My hand is covered in my own spit, I'm developing tennis elbow and possibly carpal tunnel syndrome; but on the bright side he's telling me he's almost there. I know that means I'm gonna be on my knees for another 10 minutes, but I need all the positive reinforcement I can get.

[moments of sucking that dick like there's no tomorrow]

It's coming. I mean, *he's* coming. Like right no—oh, that's…well, it's not water, but I'll take it.

25

A Real Mouthful: 100 Wacky Ways To Say 'Blowjob'

Jim Goad

1. Addressing the Court

2. BJ

3. Bagpiping

4. Basket Lunch

5. Beej

6. Blowie

7. Blowing the Love Whistle

8. Bobbing for Apples

9. Bone-Lipping

10. Buccal Onanism

11. Brentwood Hello

12. Charming the Snake

13. Climbing the Corporate Ladder

14. Cock-Gobbling

15. Copping a Doodle

16. Courting the Gay Vote

17. Drinking a Slurpee

18. Dropping on It

19. Earning your Keep

20. Essin' the Dee

21. Face-Frosting

22. Fellatio

23. Fluting

24. French Abortion

25. Gator Mouth

26. Getting a Facial

27. Getting a Lewinsky

28. Getting a Throat Culture

29. Getting to the Cream Filling

30. Giving Cone

31. Giving Face

32. Giving Head

33. Gobbling Pork

34. Going Down

35. Gumming the Root

36. Punching

37. Giving Big Jim and the Twins a Bath

38. Giving Brain

39. Giving Head

40. Gum-Rooting

41. Gumming the Green Bean

42. Head Job

43. Honkin' Bobo

44. Huffing Bone

45. Hummer

46. Interrogating the Prisoner

47. Kneeling at the Altar

48. Knob Job

49. Larking

50. Laying Some Lip

51. Licking the Lollipop

52. Making Mouth Music

53. Making the Blind See

54. Meeting with Mr. One-Eye

55. Mouth-Fucking

56. Mouth-Holstering the Nightstick

57. Mouth-Milking

58. Mouth-to-Junk Resuscitation

59. Opening Wide for Dr. Chunky

60. Oral Sodomy

61. Peeling the Banana

62. Penilingus

63. Piston Job

64. Playing Pan's Pipes

65. Playing the Pink Oboe

66. Playing the Skin Flute

67. Pole-Smoking

68. Polishing the Trailer Hitch

69. Pricknicking

70. Protein Milkshake

71. Receiving Holy Communion

72. Respecting Your Superiors

73. Sampling the Sausage

74. Scooby-Snacking

75. Secretarial Duties

76. Singing to the Choir

77. Skull-Buggery

78. Skull-Fucking

79. Slobbin' the Knob

80. Smiling at Mr. Winky

81. Smoking the Pink Pipe

82. Smoking Pole

83. Southern France

84. Speaking into the Bonophone

85. Speaking Low Genitals

86. Spit-Shining a Baseball Bat

87. Spraying the Tonsils

88. Sucking Off

89. Sucky-Ducky

90. Suck-Starting the Harley

91. Swallowing the Baloney Pony

92. Sword-Swallowing

93. Taking One's Temp with a Meat Thermometer

94. Talking into the Mic

95. Telling it to the Judge

96. Waxing the Carrot

97. Worshiping At the Altar

98. Wringing It Dry

99. Yaffling the Yogurt Cannon

100. Zipper Dinner

26

Giving My First Blowjob

Phoenix Askani

I gave my very first blowjob when I was 17 years old. He was my age and we hardly knew each other. I'm actually pretty sure we met through MySpace, but let's not talk about that. We went to a *Degrassi* signing at the mall before going back to my house to watch *The Life Aquatic*. Yes, this is a true story. We started making out after the movie on my couch, and I realized we should probably go to my bedroom because I think my mom was going to be coming home or something. He started to feel me up and my shirt came off. I felt excited because I hadn't gone very far with a guy before (but I had given one handjob and been fingered by a girl) and I had a feeling I was going to move forward at this point. I wasn't ready to lose my virginity, but I was ready to explore a little.

My mom yells from the kitchen for me to come out. I throw my shirt back on, accidentally inside out, and I go tell her "It's okay we are just talking and cuddling" when I see the concerned look on her face. She said she didn't like that we were in my room with the door closed and I should know better. She quickly but calmly suggested we go for a nice walk through the neighborhood, so I told him we should go around the block. Somehow I knew we'd just find a spot to keep making out on our "walk."

As it turned out, we made it around the corner and around the fence, right back onto my parents' property and into the backyard. There was still one of those swing set fort things standing in the middle of the yard and it was far enough from any windows and doors and concealed enough to get a little frisky in. Things got a little more heated and I decided this was the first time I'd go down on a guy. I wasn't exactly sure what I was doing but I had seen videos before. He was communicative and I just kept trying new things and reading his responses. He asked me to spit on it. I looked up at him with my almost-innocent blue eyes and did as he requested. He titty-fucked me a little bit and I'd never done that before, either. It felt awkward but I was turned on by the fact that my boobs were big enough and that he was into it. Pleasing him pleased me.

I worked his cock with my lips, hands, and tongue until he came in my mouth. I remember feeling kind of dirty and liking it. This whole sucking dick thing was new to me but I enjoyed it. A check mark appeared in an imaginary box next to BLOWJOBS in my head. To clarify detail and see if he remembered anything more than I did, I gave this old friend a call today. He remembers it vividly, saying "You don't exactly forget getting a blow job from a girl... that now does porn. You just don't." We laughed and he said, "I remember being blown away. Pun intended, I guess." I'm amused by the fact that this eight-year-old blow job will probably not be forgotten any time soon by either of us.

A month later, I ended up blowing almost an entire band in their van while it was moving. By that point, I realized I liked it more than just a little bit. It wasn't about being a sex object or being turned on by the idea of feeling a little degraded, it was about how much I wanted to get someone off. Looking back, I'm not the least bit shocked I ended up wanting to do porn.

Thought Catalog After Dark

thoughtcatalog.com/tag/after-dark/

Social

facebook.com/thoughtcatalog.afterdark
twitter.com/thoughtcatalog
tumblr.com/thoughtcatalog
instagram.com/thoughtcatalog

Corporate

www.thought.is

www.ingramcontent.com/pod-product-compliance
Lightning Source LLC
Chambersburg PA
CBHW050453290526
45786CB00006B/2282